# A Guide to
# Paracelsus Biological Medicine

# A Guide to
# Paracelsus Biological Medicine

*A new approach to health and well-being that combines noninvasive medical technology with the body's natural healing power.*

PARACELSUS BIOLOGICAL MEDICINE NETWORK

*Marion Institute • Marion, Massachusetts*

*2008*

Although the author and publisher have exhaustively researched all sources to ensure the accuracy and completeness of the information contained in this book, we assume no responsibility for errors, inaccuracies, omissions, or any inconsistency herein. Any inaccurate characterizations of people, places, or organizations are unintentional.

The information and procedures contained in this book are based on the research and the professional experience of the work of Dr. Thomas Rau at the Paracelsus Clinic. This book has been published for information and reference uses only. It is not intended in any respect as a substitute for a visit to a qualified physician or other licensed health care practitioner. Every individual is genetically different, and no method of treatment is useful for everyone. If you have a medical problem, please consult a qualified physician or health care provider for diagnosis and treatment under their supervision. The publishers and author are not responsible for any adverse effects or consequences resulting from the use of any suggestions, procedures, techniques, protocols, remedies, or preparations discussed in this book.

*Paracelsus Biological Medicine Network*
Marion Institute
202 Spring Street
Marion, Massachusetts 02738

ISBN: 978-1-60725-129-3
First Edition ISBN: 1-931188-06-8

# Contents

# Preface

## Nathaniel's Story

*In 1993, when our son Nathaniel was about to turn 13, he was diagnosed with leukemia. His rapidly deteriorating condition required three rounds of chemotherapy, followed by a bone-marrow transplant from his sister. Complications from the transplant reduced his lung capacity by 50 percent. Essentially, the cancer was in remission, but we were told that his lung capacity would not recover.*

*We began to search for alternative treatments to reverse Nathaniel's loss of function, and we read about the Paracelsus Clinic in Switzerland. We spoke with the clinic director, Dr. Thomas Rau, a pioneer of European biological medicine.*

*When Nathaniel was well enough to travel, we took him to the clinic. Five years after that initial visit, Nathaniel is a college senior leading a normal, active life, with 97 percent of his lung capacity.*

*We are confident that Paracelsus Biological Medicine, with its emphasis on noninvasive diagnostic and treatment methods and the natural healing power of the body, is the principal reason for the remission of Nathaniel's disease and his current well-being.*

*Margie Baldwin, 2002*
*Marion, Massachusetts*

## Biological medicine

Biological medicine (sometimes called European biological medicine because of its origins) is the world's most complete model of holistic medicine.

> HOLISTIC MEDICINE: an approach to medicine that assumes that the human being is a functioning system operating in a "state of wholeness." Holistic medicine views all aspects of an individual — physical, mental, emotional, and spiritual — as interrelated. Any imbalance or disharmony is thought to cause sickness. The goal of holistic medicine is to correct the imbalance and restore "wholeness."

The basic approach to biological medicine is expressed in its name: *bio* (life) and *logical* (relating to knowledge). The foundation of biological medicine is the body's own "knowledge of life" — the body's innate wisdom regarding natural life forces within and around the individual.

In biological medicine, the practitioner and the individual work together to free the body's own natural healing systems. Also, because every person is unique, biological medicine treats the *individual*, not merely the disease and its symptoms.

## Alternative medicine

Biological medicine is a form of alternative medicine. An increasing volume of information about alternative methods is entering mainstream American culture. For example, the two-volume *Health and Wellness Library* by Time-Life Books devotes nearly 200 pages to alternative medicine, and the American Medical Association (AMA) is encouraging member physicians to become better informed regarding alternative medicine and to participate in appropriate studies.*

Still, many people are not getting the facts they need in order to make some very important decisions about their own health care. This lack of knowledge, plus anxiety associated with entering new and unfamiliar territory, often creates a reluctance to explore biological medicine and other alternative health care methods. This is why it is important to answer some basic questions about biological medicine, which this guide does.

Biological medicine may not provide solutions for everyone's health care problems, but its essential philosophies and principles are sound and proven by the experiences of countless patients and practitioners, some of whom share their stories in these pages.

Ultimately, only you can determine if biological medicine makes sense for you, now or in the future. We simply hope that the information presented here will help you make better-informed decisions about your own health care and the health care needs of your loved ones.

## Paracelsus Biological Medicine

Paracelsus Biological Medicine (PBM) is a highly sophisticated scientific, holistic medical philosophy developed by Dr. Thomas Rau of the Paracelsus Clinic in Lustmühle, Switzerland.

When you are not feeling well or show symptoms of disease, you quite naturally want to feel as comfortable and confident as possible with your choice of physician and method of treatment. With this in mind, this book will help you explore PBM as an alternative approach to personal health and long-term well-being.

* AMA Resolution #514, "Alternative (Complementary) Medicine," Reference Committee E, pp. 10–11.

## About this book

This book is designed for individuals who are considering Paracelsus Biological Medicine (PBM) as a health care option or who are interested in increasing their knowledge of health care alternatives.

Its four chapters are designed to provide useful information about PBM:

- Chapter 1: Overview of Paracelsus Biological Medicine explains the concepts behind PBM and compares it with conventional medicine.

- Chapter 2: The Practice of Paracelsus Biological Medicine provides information about the professionals who observe and practice the principles of PBM.

- Chapter 3: A Closer Look at Diagnostic and Treatment Methods discusses the methods practitioners use to diagnose and treat sickness.

- Chapter 4: Patient Perspectives profiles five individuals who share their personal experiences regarding the benefits of PBM.

The book concludes with a summary of factors to consider before you try PBM.

See the glossary for key terms and the appendices for profiles of the Marion Institute and Paracelsus Biological Medicine Network, the Paracelsus Clinic, and a list of resources you may wish to consult as you continue your journey.

# Acknowledgments

The Marion Institute would like to acknowledge the following individuals:

*Thomas Rau, M.D.,* the leader of Paracelsus Biological Medicine, for helping to enhance the lives of so many patients and making all of this possible.

*Jay Frost,* a veteran medical writer, for preparing the manuscript, completing interviews, and editing the comments of others.

*Barbara Christian* and *Mike Henkle* for managing the project.

*Dede Cummings* for designing the first edition of the book and *Pixels & Pulp* for designing the second edition.

We especially acknowledge all of those who contributed financially to help bring this document to publication:

*Marion Institute*
*Paracelsus Clinic*
*Michael and Margie Baldwin*
*David and Laurie Barrett*
*Chrissie and Charlie Bascom*
*Joan Brady*
*Johnnie and Buff Chace*
*Tim Cowles*

*Milo Fay*
*Peter and Lorraine Lieberson*
*M. Whitney and Phillip Long*
*John and Joan Lundberg*
*William and Elizabeth Oates*
*Phyllis Sondes*
*John and Gerry Tuten*

# Introduction

**Welcome to the world of Paracelsus Biological Medicine!**

Chances are, you are already familiar with the concepts of Paracelsus Biological Medicine (PBM), although you may not have heard the term. You may even have received health care that is consistent with the principles of PBM.

This is because PBM combines some very *traditional* forms of health care (e.g., homeopathy, naturopathy, Chinese traditional medicine) with aspects of contemporary medical practice and technology. The result is a truly integrated form of modern medicine that is well suited for everyone, regardless of age and health care history.

As you read this primer, you will learn that PBM:

- enhances quality of life

- produces desirable outcomes in a broad range of acute and chronic illnesses

- is useful for both healing and preventative health care

- can be cost-effective by producing desirable long-term outcomes and keeping patients out of doctors' offices, hospitals, and surgery wards

- is safe for adults and children

- is generally noninvasive (i.e., minimizes the medical need for invasive procedures such as surgery or radiation therapy)

- addresses long-term psychological and behavioral disorders (e.g., anxiety, depression, substance abuse, attention deficit disorder in children and adults)

Essentially, PBM integrates the following concepts into medical practice:

- All functions in a human being are dynamic, and all organs have the capability to rebuild themselves (at least to some extent) during a lifetime.

- We are all part of nature and intensely connected to nature, mainly through nutrition, which determines our "inner milieu."

- PBM never treats diagnoses, but rather individuals; it rarely targets organs, but rather all of the body's functional systems.

- PBM requires new ways of thinking about one's health — a belief that all disease has a purpose and that symptoms are never "diseases" per se, but rather signs that the body's regulation is out of sync. (This relates to the fact that we are all part of nature and respond in a natural manner to internal and external events).

Perhaps most important for many patients, PBM is *safe*. It features comprehensive detoxification and stimulation techniques that rarely, if ever, cause side effects or peripheral damage to the body (such as might occur with chemotherapy or other aggressive treatments in conventional medicine).

Keep in mind that PBM can be effectively combined with conventional Western (or "allopathic") medical practices, often enhancing outcomes. This has been dramatically demonstrated in patients with cardiovascular disease, chronic inflammatory diseases (such as rheumatoid arthritis), and even severe cancers.

As you will learn, PBM is logical, is easy to understand, and treats patients as individuals. However, learning about PBM — and applying its principles in one's own life — involves change. Change begins with knowledge, and this primer is an excellent starting point to develop that knowledge.

*Dr. Thomas M. Rau*
Chief Medical Director
Paracelsus Clinic
Lustmühle, Switzerland

# Chapter 1
# Overview of
# Paracelsus Biological Medicine

### What is Paracelsus Biological Medicine?

As suggested in the preface, Paracelsus Biological Medicine (PBM) utilizes a holistic approach to health and wellness that allows the human body to maximize its own innate healing powers.

A good way to understand PBM is to consider the methods conventional — or *allopathic* — physicians use to diagnose and treat disease, then compare those methods with the practice of PBM.

In general, conventional physicians are trained to identify symptoms of disease and to recommend treatments that eliminate or alleviate those symptoms. This approach often makes the patient feel better, but may not "cure" the disease or address the underlying condition(s) that allow the disease to manifest in the first place.

> ALLOPATHIC: a system of therapeutics in which diseases are treated by producing a condition that is incompatible with or antagonistic to the disease and its symptoms. Examples of allopathic treatments include prescription pharmaceuticals, radiation, and surgery. All M.D.s in the United States are licensed to practice allopathic medicine.

## Does Paracelsus Biological Medicine go beyond treating symptoms?

Yes. In addition to treating particular symptoms, PBM looks for the root causes of those symptoms. These root causes may consist of several factors that, over time, can allow disease-causing toxins to build up in the body.

These factors include:

- diet
- lifestyle
- family history
- stress
- aging
- environmental factors
- trauma
- exposure to bacteria or virus

Looked at another way, our health often relates to how we feel, live, work, play, love, relax, socialize, and so on. Physiologically and psychologically, we all have "up-building" (regenerative) and "down-grading" (degenerative) forces within us, all of which are dependent on the factors listed above.

PBM assesses the body's entire combination of physical, mental, emotional, and spiritual factors — everything that makes us tick — and tries to identify which combination of these factors may cause the body to be out of balance.

## Does Paracelsus Biological Medicine address these imbalances?

Yes, exactly. PBM practitioners are trained to identify these imbalances and recommend treatments that allow *nature* to take over and promote a restoration of balance.

These treatments support the body's "up-building" forces, help reverse degenerative activity, and promote long-term healing. They are generally noninvasive (surgery and radiation are examples of invasive treatments), and they rarely require the use of prescription drugs (which usually are not "natural" agents, often cause harmful side effects, and typically treat symptoms instead of the root causes of disease).

## Can you give an example of how conventional medicine and Paracelsus Biological Medicine might approach the same condition?

Let's take a simple example with which most of us are familiar, a child with an ear infection.

*Conventional medicine.* A conventional, allopathically trained pediatrician would normally perform the examination by checking the child's throat, listening to the lungs, and examining the ears. A typical examination might rule out flu, pneumonia, and other conditions. However, the doctor might notice swelling and redness in the child's ears and correctly diagnose an ear infection (*otitis media* in medical jargon).

In most cases, the pediatrician would prescribe an antibiotic, and perhaps recommend an analgesic or over-the-counter (OTC) cold medication to help relieve inflammation and pain. Chances are, in a day or two, the symptoms would disappear, and the child would resume normal activities.

Note that in this example the physician successfully alleviated symptoms (inflammation, pain). However, the physician also recommended the introduction of an antibiotic into the body. The drug killed the bacteria, exactly as it was supposed to do. The child, much to his or her satisfaction, experienced rapid relief from earache pain, but the antibiotic might also have destroyed millions of nonpathogenic bacteria essential for effective immune response.

Chances are, the drug actually interrupted the body's *natural* healing response. Thus, the child's immune system may not be any stronger the next time an infection occurs. This may increase the likelihood of future infections and create a dependency on antibiotics whenever the doctor suspects an infection.

NATUROPATHY: a system of medicine that treats health conditions by utilizing the body's inherent, natural ability to heal. Naturopathy aids the healing process by incorporating a variety of alternative methods based on the patient's individual needs. Diet, lifestyle, work, and personal history are all considered when determining a treatment regimen.

*Paracelsus Biological Medicine.* Now let's assume we have the same child with the same symptoms, except this time the parent takes the child to a PBM practitioner. Rather than zeroing in on symptoms, this practitioner would take a longer-term, bigger-picture assessment of the child's health.

This practitioner might use the same noninvasive diagnostic techniques to rule out serious disease, but he or she would probably spend a bit more time with the parent and child asking questions about home and school environment, the child's (and the family's) history of bacterial infections, the child's diet and historical use of antibiotics, and so on.*

---

\* It should be noted that some allopathic physicians will perform a comprehensive, detailed profile when diagnosing a patient. The point here is that virtually *all* Paracelsus Biological Medicine practitioners follow this procedure. Only in this manner can the practitioner recommend an appropriate treatment that goes beyond the rapid alleviation of symptoms.

The PBM practitioner would arrive at the same diagnosis: *otitis media*. However, instead of using the conventional "tried and true" method of prescribing an antibiotic and OTC medications, the practitioner would recommend less harmful treatments that would support and strengthen the body's natural healing power.

This practitioner would, of course, address the child's symptoms — no one wants to see a child suffer from pain. Accordingly, the practitioner might suggest a naturopathic ear oil (often available over-the-counter at retail drugstores and health food stores) to reduce pain, as well as an herbal preparation, taken orally, to promote immune stimulation.

Symptomatic relief would probably occur quickly, but the complete, natural healing response might take longer. By allowing this natural healing response to occur, PBM allows the immune system to strengthen itself, perhaps increasing resistance to future infections.

### Is Paracelsus Biological Medicine effective for more serious, chronic diseases?

Yes. PBM has an excellent track record for the successful treatment and management or elimination of serious, chronic, and potentially debilitating diseases. Asthma, allergies, diabetes, chronic fatigue syndrome, rheumatoid arthritis, depression, and even some cancers often respond to PBM.

Later in this book, you will learn more about how PBM addresses these serious diseases, sometimes in the words of patients.

| Conventional Medicine | Paracelsus Biological Medicine |
|---|---|
| • Trains practitioners as specialists who tend to view the body as made up of separate systems (cardiovascular, endocrine, nervous, etc.). | • Trains practitioners to diagnose and treat holistically, i.e., to view the human being as a whole (physically, mentally, emotionally, spiritually) and each person as an individual. |
| • Generally diagnoses specific diseases (e.g., a general practitioner for flu or pneumonia, a cardiologist for heart disease, a psychiatrist for mental health, etc.) and treats symptoms (e.g., antibiotics for infections). | • Treats the body, mind, and spirit as an integral, interrelated system. Attempts to diagnose and treat the underlying cause(s) of disease within the context of the patient's life, family, work, relationships, lifestyle, etc. |
| • Tries to cure disease from the "outside in," e.g., by introducing pharmaceuticals to the body or performing invasive procedures. | • Attempts to promote true healing from the "inside out," e.g., by promoting and supporting the body's natural healing methods. |
| • Often utilizes "standardized" methods of care (usually based on results of clinical and empirical trials and clinical practice guidelines). | • Generally develops highly individualized treatment regimens (based on a holistic diagnosis that assesses genetic factors, environment, lifestyle, etc.). |
| • Focuses on prompt relief of symptoms and accelerated cures. | • Focuses on prompt relief of symptoms and rapid cures when appropriate, but takes a longer-term, holistic approach with an eye toward genuine and permanent healing. |

## What are some other differences between Paracelsus Biological Medicine and conventional Western medicine?

Conventional medicine has historically attempted to manage the healing process by isolating, identifying, and measuring a broad range of physiological, physical, and chemical reactions that can be documented by modern science. Usually, these measurements are assessed in clinical trials, such as those that compare and contrast the effects of new pharmaceutical agents on selected patient populations.

Conventional medicine also tends to isolate the various systems of the body, sometimes focusing on one system while de-emphasizing others. These systems include the cardiovascular, nervous, endocrine, pulmonary, gastrointestinal, musculoskeletal, and reproductive systems. This is one reason why conventional medicine has so many specialist physicians — cardiologists, rheumatologists, urologists, gynecologists, endocrinologists, and so on. Critics often refer to this approach as the "reductionist" model of Western medicine.

PBM does not isolate or reduce the body into a series of discrete systems. Instead, it considers the human being as a comprehensive, integrated entity — body (and all its physiological systems, considered together), mind, spirit, and soul — and takes into account both the internal and external environments of the individual.

PBM is capable of diagnosing diseases and conditions in a very precise manner because its practitioners take the time to map the connections between every system and organ in the body.

## Do practitioners of Paracelsus Biological Medicine utilize high-tech procedures?

When appropriate, yes.

Conventional medicine places a great deal of emphasis on techniques and technology. Because PBM focuses on the inherent, natural healing power of the body, you might think that it does not utilize modern technology. This is not true.

> THERMOGRAPHY: a diagnostic technique that utilizes a thermalized (temperature-sensitive) wand, or thermister, to record skin temperature at 181 points on the body, first at standard room temperature, then at a lower temperature. Responses suggest organs and systems that are abnormally active and those that are depleted or not functioning properly.

In fact, many practitioners of PBM routinely use highly advanced noninvasive diagnostic procedures to help assess the overall performance of the body's interrelated systems. For example, a practitioner might order *computerized thermography* to evaluate the status of a patient's immune, digestive, cardiovascular, and autonomic nervous systems.

A practitioner might also take advantage of *darkfield microscopy* to assess cellular activity in the blood. This procedure magnifies live blood cells for detailed study of cell structure and function.

PBM also utilizes technology in many other ways, including dried blood tests; heart-rate variability tests; and saliva, blood, and urine analysis.

## Is Paracelsus Biological Medicine considered a form of "alternative medicine"?

Yes. There is no one- or two-sentence definition of alternative medicine that satisfies everyone but, in the United States, PBM is definitely considered a form of alternative medicine.

In fact, PBM is made up of a rich array of techniques, modalities, and medical systems that may be unfamiliar to the majority of the public and are not practiced by most "mainstream" M.D.s. Consequently, these procedures are generally considered "alternatives" to those that Americans typically experience in the delivery of health care.

## What are some examples of alternative medicine?

There are many examples. Most (but not all) come to us from other parts of the world or from ancient healing traditions — settings in which they are/were not considered "alternative" at all.

For example, the use of herbs as medicine is a centuries-old practice found all over the world. In recent decades, herbal medicines have acquired a strong presence in the United States, where they can be purchased at pharmacies and health and nutrition centers and, in some cases, prepared at home.

Two examples of alternative medicine (holistic medicine and naturopathy) were introduced earlier in this book. Other examples of alternative therapies include:

"While the term alternative medicine may conjure up some pretty exotic images, many of these therapies are more familiar than you think. If you've ever massaged your temples to ease a headache, applied an ice pack to a sprained ankle, or listened to your car radio to de-stress during a traffic jam, you've already practiced some simple natural healing techniques."

- Bill Gottlieb, *New Choices in Natural Healing*, Rodale Press, 1995, p. 4.

- **Acupressure.** Acupressure is a traditional Chinese therapeutic technique in which, using fingers or hands, pressure is applied to specific points on the body to alter the body's internal flow of life energy (referred to as "chi"), strengthening it, calming it, reducing it, increasing it, or eliminating blockages.

- **Acupuncture.** This is another traditional Chinese technique. With acupuncture, the flow of chi is released by the insertion of hair-thin needles at specific points on the body. Both acupuncture and acupressure are based on the traditional Chinese theory of meridians (see box).

> MERIDIANS: According to traditional Chinese medicine, acupressure and acupuncture points are aligned along 14 energetic pathways within the body. These pathways are often called meridians.
>
> Twelve of the meridians are bilateral (identical pathways on both sides of the body), and the other two are unilateral (running along the midline of the body).
>
> Meridians do not correspond in any known way to the various anatomical and physiological principles taught in Western medical schools.
>
> Practitioners of PBM often incorporate the meridian theory into their methods. For example, it is not unusual for a practitioner to successfully treat an intestinal dysfunction by repairing or removing a tooth that lies in the same meridian as the large intestine.

- **Ayurvedic medicine.** Ayurvedic* theory suggests that diseases of the body are caused by stresses in the awareness, or consciousness, of the individual. These stresses lead to unhealthy practices, producing ill health. Treatments in ayurvedic medicine, which originated in India more than 5,000 years ago, include yoga-related body postures, breathing exercises, meditative techniques, special diets, and herbal remedies.

- **Homeopathy.** Homeopathy is a therapeutic system in which diseases are treated by substances that can cause symptoms of disease in a healthy person but that, when administered in minute doses, can cure those same symptoms. Most homeopaths practice constitutional homeopathy, a holistic approach that assumes that each person's "constitu-

---

\* Interestingly, the term *ayurveda* derives from the Indian words meaning "life" and "knowledge." You'll recall that "biological" comes from the same root words (derived from Latin).

tion" (physical, emotional, and mental factors) should be addressed in order to heal the disease.

- **Osteopathy.** Osteopathy focuses on addressing problems in the musculoskeletal system to correct and improve the general functioning of the body. A doctor of osteopathy (D.O.) combines manipulation of the joints, physical therapy, and recommendations for correcting posture. As a holistic form of health care, osteopathy also addresses emotional and psychological factors, nutrition, and lifestyle when addressing sickness and promoting good health.

- **Traditional Chinese medicine.** Traditional Chinese medicine is an ancient system of holistic health care that uses a variety of treatments including acupressure, acupuncture, herbal therapies, and massage, along with health-sustaining energetic body movement such as *tai chi*. Like biological medicine and many other alternative health care methods, Chinese medicine takes a holistic approach to health care by treating the entire body rather than individual systems.

Paracelsus Biological Medicine (PBM) synthesizes components of these (and sometimes other) forms of alternative medicine and combines these methods with modern, high-tech, noninvasive procedures.

## Does Paracelsus Biological Medicine apply to dental health, too?

Yes. While allopathic medicine generally views teeth as separate from the rest of the body and unrelated to overall health, dental treatment is often an essential element of PBM.

Root canals, implants, and dental amalgams (fillings) may contain heavy metals that can affect brain cells and the nervous system. Many of us have dental amalgams composed of toxic substances like mercury (which is so toxic that dentists must dispose of it as a hazardous waste) and palladium. In PBM, the removal of these amalgams from the mouth helps free the body of these toxins and is a fundamental part of the healing process.

Using a Panorex (a high-tech procedure that provides a detailed, panoramic picture of the teeth and entire jaw), PBM practitioners can obtain crucial information about the overall state of a person's health.

IS PBM SAFE? Yes. In fact, most PBM practitioners and their patients consider Paracelsus Biological Medicine to be safer than conventional medicine. This is because PBM generally avoids the use of invasive procedures (such as surgery) and the use of mainstream prescription pharmaceuticals (which may introduce chemicals and toxins that do not naturally occur in the body and cause uncomfortable side effects).

In cases where surgery is required, pre- and post-operative procedures may be performed using PBM principles. For example, practitioners of PBM do not recommend the use of metal staples (which may introduce toxic substances into the body and restrict energy flow) to close incisions.

## How important is the removal of toxins in Paracelsus Biological Medicine?

Very important. This becomes easier to understand when you consider the body as a "disease barrel." This analogy, developed by Dr. Thomas Rau, a pioneer of Paracelsus Biological Medicine, compares the human body's susceptibility to disease with an ordinary waste barrel. This is our "disease barrel."

Our body has the ability to accept and respond to an enormous variety of stresses and toxins. However, if allowed to accumulate,

## The Disease Barrel
To understand the reasons for the development of chronic diseases

Acute disease released by:

Endobiontic load
Disturbance foci
Trace element deficiency
Toxic load
Heavy metals
Hyperacidity
Protein excess
Geopathic disturbance
Miasmatic load
Constitution/genetics

Life of stresses and toxins

Illness is a state of imbalance. An individual's "disease barrel" fills up over time until eventually it overflows and manifests as an acute (short-term) illness, a chronic (long-term) condition, or even a life-threatening disease such as cancer. Biological medicine helps to empty out the "disease barrel," promoting short-term healing and long-term well-being.

© 1997 by Dr. Thomas Rau, Paracelsus Klink, Lustmühle, Switzerland

these factors can exceed the body's ability to handle them. When this happens, the body's natural balancing system (called "homeostasis") becomes compromised.

Put simply, illness is a state of imbalance. As Dr. Rau states, an individual's disease barrel fills up over time until eventually it overflows and manifests as an acute (short-term) illness, a chronic (long-term) condition, or even a life-threatening disease such as cancer. PBM helps to empty out the disease barrel, promoting short-term healing and long-term well-being.

## What specific acute and chronic illnesses can be treated with Paracelsus Biological Medicine?

The holistic PBM model is suitable for the treatment of many acute and virtually all chronic diseases, including:

- allergies (including hidden food or environmental allergies)
- asthma
- cancer and tumor diseases
- cardiovascular disease (including angina pectoris and hypertension)
- chronic fatigue syndrome
- fungal infections (e.g., candidiasis)
- hay fever
- immunosuppressive disorders
- intoxication and amalgam problems
- neuralgias
- neurodermatitis
- rheumatoid arthritis
- allergic rhinitis
- stomach and colon disorders (e.g., colitis, constipation, Crohn's disease, diarrhea, digestive problems, flatulence, ulcers)
- tooth and jaw infections

## Is Paracelsus Biological Medicine appropriate for children?

Acute and chronic disease and behavioral disorders of children can be treated effectively and gently by PBM. Children are very often highly responsive to the natural approaches of PBM.

## How can I be confident that Paracelsus Biological Medicine works?

No system of medicine can guarantee success for every condition in every patient. What works for one person may be less effective for another. Each system — conventional or alternative — is well suited to address certain health care conditions.

In PBM, an individual's willingness to take responsibility for his or her own healing is part of the process. Consequently, it is important to be well-informed.

We hope that the principles outlined in this guidebook will help you make appropriate choices for your particular situation.

When the crisis of disease occurs, conventional medical procedures often zero in to eradicate symptoms, not to eliminate the causes. While this approach has an important place — and is indeed essential — in the menu of health care options, Paracelsus Biological Medicine strongly asserts that unless the causes are addressed, crises will recur, as we see in chronic diseases such as asthma, cardiovascular disease, rheumatoid arthritis, and even cancer.

## Chapter 2
# The Practice of
# Paracelsus Biological Medicine

### Who practices Paracelsus Biological Medicine?

A variety of health care professionals practice Paracelsus Biological Medicine (PBM).

Keep in mind that PBM is not considered a medical specialty in the same sense that we think of family practice, cardiology, gastroenterology, urology, and other medical disciplines as specialties.

The fact is, virtually all types of practitioners can incorporate the principles of PBM into their practices. A variety of health care professionals — including conventional physicians, chiropractors, dentists, doctors of osteopathy and homeopathy, and nurse practitioners — can use techniques of PBM when diagnosing and treating patients.

### Are these professionals licensed to practice Paracelsus Biological Medicine?

There is currently no special licensing requirement for the incorporation of PBM in medical practice.

Medical practitioners are licensed to practice in their individual disciplines by appropriate licensing boards and professional accreditation organizations. For example, a general practitioner must be licensed in general practice (or family medicine), and an obstetrician-gynecologist (ob-gyn) must be licensed by the appropriate ob-gyn licensing board. In the United States, most medical licensing is performed at the state level — each of the 50 states has its own licensing boards.

If you have any concerns about the qualifications of any medical practitioner, you should investigate his or her background and be aware of any licensing requirements in your state or county. Ask for detailed information about diagnostic methods, treatments, and procedures the practitioner uses, and remember that you are in charge of decisions about your own health care.

### Are practitioners of Paracelsus Biological Medicine required to have any special kind of formal training in biological medicine?

Medical professionals can incorporate whatever degree of PBM they feel comfortable with into their practices, and anyone who utilizes principles of PBM should have some formal training that meets their individual requirements and professional goals.

Formal training and certification in PBM is currently available at the Paracelsus Clinic in Switzerland. Periodically, training programs are offered in the USA through the Paracelsus Biological Medicine Network (PBMN). Visit www.pbmn.org for more information. For international trainings, please visit www.paracelsus.ch.

## Are practitioners of Paracelsus Biological Medicine graduates of medical school?

Some are. All licensed physicians (M.D.s) who treat patients in the United States are graduates of accredited medical schools, regardless of whether or not they utilize PBM methods.

Other medical professionals (i.e., non physicians, such as psychologists, chiropractors, physician assistants, and nurse practitioners) who use biological medicine techniques in their practices must possess accreditation credentials issued by the appropriate licensing boards in their specific disciplines.

> TRAINING AND CERTIFICATION IN PARACELSUS BIOLOGICAL MEDICINE: To further the understanding and practice of PBM, the Marion Institute has held training seminars for practitioners and created the Paracelsus Biological Medicine Network (PBMN). Many U.S. practitioners have completed the Marion Institute's two-year certification program in biological medicine and are affiliated with the PBMN.

## Where can I find a practitioner of Paracelsus Biological Medicine?

There are several hundred physicians and other practitioners in the United States who currently incorporate PBM principles into their practices.

If a health care provider gave you this publication, chances are that he or she uses PBM methods or knows someone who does.

For information about where to find a practitioner of PBM in your area, consult Appendix A at the back of this book or visit www.pbmn.org.

## Can I consult a practitioner of Paracelsus Biological Medicine and still continue to see my personal physician?

Yes. If you are considering PBM as an alternative or complement to the care you currently receive, we recommend that you share your thoughts and health care goals with your personal physician. Tell your physician about the options you are considering.

A dedicated physician will support your efforts to learn more about PBM and other types of alternative health care (see box below). In some cases, your personal physician may even refer you to a professional who is familiar with PBM.

---

ONE PHYSICIAN'S OPINION: "In my work as a physician — and as a practitioner of alternative medicine — I am constantly reminded of the importance of keeping an open mind when it comes to finding out what's best for my patients. Years of experience have shown me that no single approach to health care has all the answers; the search for healing solutions often requires a willingness to look beyond one remedy or system of treatment.

"At the same time, I also feel a deep responsibility to be selective — to recognize important distinctions among the vast array of treatment options available. Because the same therapy can affect different patients in different ways, an approach that works for one patient may do nothing for another.

"My job, then, is not just to seek out which remedies are available or safe, but to prescribe the course of treatment that best suits the patient's condition and lifestyle. I've discovered, though, that I can't do this job alone. Whatever the therapy, patients respond dramatically better to treatment when they take an active, confident role in their own health care."*

- Jeffrey Midgow, M.D.

* *Health and Wellness*, The Southwestern Company, 2000, p.8
  ©Time Life Inc.

---

For most individuals, PBM is not an either/or proposition. PBM offers an alternative to conventional medicine, often in a complementary manner.

It is up to you to decide the extent to which you want to use PBM — to treat a specific disease or condition or to incorporate PBM into your life on a long-term basis.

## Are consultations and treatments in Paracelsus Biological Medicine covered by health insurance or managed care plans?

Possibly. It depends on the state you live in and your insurance plan. A few states and many health plans are expanding coverage to include some types of alternative health care.

In many situations, health plans require that treatment for alternative medicine be defined as "medically necessary." Usually, a conventional physician, who functions as a "gatekeeper," decides what particular treatment is medically necessary. Keep in mind that some physicians who determine medical necessity may be biased against some alternative medicine practices.

Recently, in response to consumer demand, as well as to evidence that alternative medicine works for many people, coverage for alternative health care options has become more common.

If you are considering PBM and are concerned about insurance coverage, ask your practitioner if he or she has experience with your particular insurer regarding reimbursement for alternative health care. If the answer is no, contact your health insurance representative and obtain current information about possible coverage for alternative medical treatments.

Be specific about any preventive measures, diagnostic procedures, and treatments that you are thinking about. If it turns out that your plan does not cover these items, it may be worth your time and money to shop around for a different insurance plan. You may find a plan that is better suited for your health care needs. If you are unsuccessful in your efforts to obtain coverage, you will be required to pay out-of-pocket for expenses associated with PBM.

## Chapter 3
# A Closer Look at Diagnostic and Treatment Methods

**How does a practitioner of Paracelsus Biological Medicine diagnose disease or other ailments?**

As mentioned earlier, Paracelsus Biological Medicine (PBM) takes a holistic view of the human body and does not isolate or reduce the body into separate systems. Thus, an assessment of the functioning of each of the body's systems is essential to diagnosis. Based upon this information, treatments are designed to help revitalize organs and systems so that the individual can *resist* disease and prevent recurrences.

**Isn't this the same thing that conventional and holistic practitioners do?**

To an extent, yes, but PBM is different. Conventional medicine is designed to identify disease and treat symptoms. Rarely, however, do conventional physicians — and even practitioners of holistic medicine — attempt to detect subtle systemic imbalances that can predict major illness. Most practitioners of PBM take the time to do this.

### What diagnostic techniques does the practitioner use to identify these subtle imbalances?

The practitioner usually begins with a comprehensive interview, a physical examination, and selected medical tests.

Tests may include pulse reading; analyses of blood, urine, and saliva; dental and skin examinations; hearing and vision tests; cardiovascular tests; kinesthetic evaluation (see box); and others.

KINESTHETICS: Kinesthetics refers to the science of movement. In biological medicine, a practitioner often assesses the ways in which a patient perceives movement, weight, position, etc. The purpose is to identify changes in the angles of joints, which may be indicative of disease.

Together, the interview, exam, and tests enable the practitioner to customize a treatment program that matches your individual needs.

Generally, you can expect a PBM practitioner to conduct what is sometimes called a "biological terrain assessment" during diagnosis.

A terrain assessment evaluates the health status of an individual through analysis of the blood, urine, and saliva.

### What are some of the specific diagnostic measures used in the "terrain assessment"?

A terrain assessment evaluates the health status of an individual through analysis of the blood, urine, and saliva. Prior to the tests, a patient is asked to fast for 12 hours — avoiding even toothpaste and the use of cosmetics before the tests are administered.

Practitioners use the results of these tests to determine how well the body absorbs nutrients and produces energy. While these tests do not identify specific diseases, they can provide an excellent profile of overall health. Blood tests can help determine the presence of environmental toxins in the body. Analysis of saliva reveals information about liver function. Urinalysis reveals the level of kidney function and the ability of the kidneys to filter toxins from the body.

Other diagnostic measures might include computerized thermography and darkfield microscopy (both described in chapter 1).

## How does Paracelsus Biological Medicine attempt to restore health?

For the practitioner of PBM, helping to restore a patient's health is a threefold process:

1. The practitioner performs an appropriate combination of diagnostic tests to identify blockages, imbalances, and potential toxins.

2. The practitioner works with the patient to develop treatments that systematically remove stored toxins that may be obstructing energy flow and the balance among systems and organs.

3. The practitioner recommends treatments, dietary changes, lifestyle alterations, etc., that will help stimulate the responsiveness of all the body's systems or calm and balance overactive systems.

## Can you provide an example?

The following is an excellent example provided by a patient who suffered from chronic asthma.

A PATIENT'S STORY: I was incapacitated by my asthma for nearly six years. I slept 20 hours a day and took six different medications three times a day, all to no avail. Finally, I sought out the care of a practitioner of Paracelsus Biological Medicine.

When you go to see a PBM practitioner, you talk about *everything* that's affecting you. My doctor spent hours talking with me, not just minutes like other doctors. The doctor ordered a computerized thermography to assess how well my immune, digestive, autonomic nervous, and circulatory systems were functioning. A technician measured about 100 points on my body, first at normal room temperature, then in a cooler room, to determine how my skin, nervous system, and corresponding organs were functioning. These responses reflected where my body's functions were impaired, and, in my case, my liver and adrenal functions registered as weak.

Next, the doctor looked at my blood through a darkfield microscope, a remarkable German invention that shows live blood cells against a dark background, which allows a close look at cell activity. He noticed that my white blood cells were sluggish, suggesting an impaired immune system.

The diagnosis? Food allergies.

I was advised to eliminate wheat and dairy products from my diet and to apply castor oil packs to my liver — a naturopathic treatment — at home. He also prescribed naturopathic remedies to help detoxify my liver and revitalize my adrenal glands.

Over the next six months, I was able to reduce and finally eliminate my asthma medications. Today, I have enough energy to work full days in my restaurant business, baby-sit my grandchildren in the evening, and bake wheat-free breads and rolls for my on-line business.

**The previous example is for an asthma patient. What if I were diagnosed with another disease, say, diabetes or even cancer?**

The principles are the same, although the practitioner will develop specific diagnostic procedures and treatments that match the unique needs of each patient. Chapter 4 describes the experiences of patients with different diseases, including cancer.

**What if I have a relatively simple ailment, such as the common cold, a seasonal flu, or an upper-respiratory infection? Is Paracelsus Biological Medicine appropriate?**

PBM can help reduce the frequency of these events or help prevent them altogether. PBM remedies can help alleviate the symptoms of many acute and chronic ailments.

Keep in mind, however, that certain common ailments, such as the common cold, represent a natural way to rid the body of harmful organisms and *strengthen the immune system*. In these cases, most PBM practitioners will take a longer-term view by addressing symptoms while allowing the body's natural healing process to take its own course.

**What treatment methods are used by practitioners of Paracelsus Biological Medicine?**

Let's take a closer look at some of the treatment methods commonly used in PBM:

## Homeopathy

Homeopathy (introduced in chapter 1) is an inexpensive, nontoxic system of medicine used by hundreds of millions of people worldwide. It is especially effective for treating chronic illnesses that fail to respond to conventional treatment. Homeopathic methods are well suited for self-care for conditions such as the common cold and flu.

Homeopathy is a method of healing based on the idea that "like cures like." In other words, an agent that might cause certain symptoms of illness in a healthy person can cure the same symptoms in someone who is sick.

Homeopathic remedies are derived from plant, mineral, and animal extracts that are highly diluted using precise methods that eliminate toxicity while increasing a substance's potential to relieve symptoms or cure disease.

Homeopathic remedies are most effective in the treatment of ailments that have not yet caused severe damage to body organs and systems and for conditions that require the chronic use of conventional pharmaceuticals. Allergies and arthritis are two examples of these conditions.

In the United States, homeopathic remedies are acknowledged and regulated by the federal Food and Drug Administration. Many remedies are available over the counter at retail pharmacies, while some must be prescribed by a licensed practitioner.

TESTING HOMEOPATHIC REMEDIES: Most homeopathic remedies have been evaluated in medical trials in which healthy subjects receive undiluted or slightly diluted doses of substances known to cause sickness.

During the tests, clinicians assess the subjects' physical, mental, and emotional responses to determine the range of symptoms produced by the substance.

Responses have been recorded over many years and published in a reference document that provides homeopathic practitioners with evidence for their decision-making.

## Ayurvedic medicine

The primary focus of ayurvedic medicine is preventive health care, although ayurvedic methods can provide relief for many chronic ailments. Medical researchers are currently studying the effects of ayurvedic treatments for arthritis, cancer, high cholesterol, Parkinson's disease, diabetes, and chemical addictions.

Ayurvedic practitioners use a variety of treatments and methods for healing, which are usually separated into two categories: constitutional and therapeutic. Constitutional treatments involve lifestyle changes, breathing exercises, and adjustments to sleeping and eating habits. A practitioner may also recommend dietary changes that include certain herbal supplements.

## Chiropractic

Like other aspects of Paracelsus Biological Medicine, chiropractic care assumes that the body has an innate self-healing ability and always seeks homeostasis. Chiropractic theory holds that the central nervous system plays a key role in maintaining homeostasis, but that certain misalignments of the joints or irregularities of motion can interfere with nervous system activity, causing pain and possible deterioration of general health. By manipulating muscles and joints — especially the spine — chiropractors readjust these irregularities, enhancing neuromuscular function and restoring homeostasis.

Until recently, chiropractic was considered a form of alternative medicine. In recent years, chiropractic has gained wide acceptance in the United States. Chiropractic services are now covered by Medicare and most major insurance and managed care plans.

Chiropractic care is considered beneficial in the treatment of arthritis, asthma, back pain, repetitive motion disorders (e.g., carpal tunnel syndrome), chronic fatigue syndrome, headache, tendonitis, and many other common ailments.

## Neural therapy

Neural therapy involves the injection of homeopathic remedies into the body's acupuncture points. The remedies are introduced into the body's autonomic nervous system, which regulates all involuntary bodily functions (such as heartbeat and respiration). The autonomic nervous system features sensors throughout the skin, and thus provides pathways for the delivery of medicine to the body's key organs and systems.

In PBM, practitioners use a mild anesthetic (e.g., lidocaine or procaine) as the basic ingredient in an injection, adding one or more homeopathic or other natural remedies, selected by the practitioner, according to the diagnosis.

The injection points are carefully identified according to sources of blockage or disturbance diagnosed by the practitioner. For example, injecting lung points can help address asthma or lung disorders, while injecting certain bladder or kidney points can help enhance adrenal output and improve kidney function.

## What role does dentistry play in Paracelsus Biological Medicine?

Conventional medicine has arbitrarily separated dentistry from medicine — an unusual distinction, since the mouth and teeth are essential parts of the body. Consequently, conventional physicians rarely consider the mouth and teeth when attempting to diagnose a problem.

On the other hand, practitioners of PBM emphasize that the mouth and teeth can have a profound impact on what occurs in other parts of the body. Because of the meridian system, each tooth connects to a specific organ or system in the body. Accordingly, an unhealthy tooth on the heart meridian could, along with other factors (such as age or poor diet), contribute to heart disease.

Consider root canals, which are widely used in modern dentistry. A completed root canal may harbor a hidden infection that can undermine the immune system by forcing it to fight a chronic, low-grade infection. The same root canal may also weaken corresponding meridian organs. Conversely, weakened organs can affect the health of a corresponding tooth, sometimes causing decay.

Consider, too, the presence of mercury, widely used in amalgam fillings. Mercury is a known poison that in many circumstances must be disposed of according to stringent requirements. Small amounts of mercury may leak from fillings and circulate throughout the body, where toxicity can cause chronic fatigue, depression, and joint pain.

PBM can identify mercury toxicity through a variety of tests. Mercury can then be removed, according to strict guidelines by a dentist trained in the procedure. In addition, PBM practitioners often recommend oral supplements that can help remove mercury from the organs and systems of the body.

The Paracelsus Clinic features dentists on staff whose services in the diagnosis and treatment of disease complement those of physicians.

## What can I do on my own to promote the healing process?

To optimize the value of your PBM treatment, it is important to follow dietary guidelines (see Dr. Rau's book, *The Swiss Secret to Optimal Health*), take appropriate supplements, follow an exercise or bodywork routine (see box), and perform other activities recommended by your practitioner.

> BODYWORK: Bodywork refers to a variety of techniques that promote relaxation and treat certain ailments, especially musculoskeletal disorders. Treatment techniques usually involve some combination of massage, movement awareness, structural realignment, and energy balancing. Most bodywork regimens take a holistic approach to care and include treatment of both mind and body.

Because PBM assumes the integration of mind and body, identifying and addressing core emotional issues are also essential for successful treatment. PBM can call upon a wide range of healing therapies that target the emotions — including homeopathy, imagery, meditation, and psychotherapy.

Gaining familiarity with the underlying theories supporting PBM will help enhance your understanding of how and why its diagnostic and treatment techniques work. You may also find it useful to learn about the experiences related by patients of PBM, such as the patients profiled in the next chapter.

# Chapter 4
# Patient Perspectives

ONE OF THE BEST WAYS to assess the value of a particular approach to medicine is to hear the first-person stories of patients. Here, in their own words, are the experiences of five individuals whose lives have been changed by Paracelsus Biological Medicine (PBM).

### Serita Winthrop, 58, *social worker, New York, N.Y. (eczema)*

I was diagnosed with eczema* when I was just three months old. As I got older, I learned that my condition was chronic — a lifelong condition that flared up periodically, always when I was under a lot of stress. I had three, month-long hospital stays at ages three, 10, and 23. That last one was three months after my first marriage, and it was at that time that I was given injections and pills of cortisone as well as creams.

It wasn't until I was 50 that I discovered I had severe osteoporosis as a result of the cortisone. When I had a severe outbreak after my second marriage, I wanted to avoid cortisone but was desperate and enormously relieved when Dr. Rau at the Paracelsus Clinic told me

---

* An inflammatory skin condition characterized by redness, itching, oozing, crusting, and scaling.

that removing the metal fillings from my teeth was very likely to help with the clearing of my eczema. He also treated the osteoporosis.

The combination of treatments that I had under care at the Paracelsus Clinic — and the addressing of emotional and spiritual issues — brought my skin under control. I am learning to listen better to my feelings, though my skin remains a barometer (I actually had to leave my second marriage in order for my skin to clear completely). It took a couple of years for the metal to leave my system, but Dr. Rau had warned me that it would take that long.

I will always feel enormous gratitude to Dr. Rau, whose intuitive powers are part of what make him a brilliant healer.

### Richard Griscom, *66, semi-retired attorney, Galisteo, N.M. (prostate cancer)*

I was undergoing a routine physical in October 1999. My PSA (prostate-specific antigen) test was normal, but my internist suspected that my prostate gland was too large and recommended a biopsy. He referred me to a specialist and, as a result of the biopsy, I was diagnosed with prostate cancer.

I consulted with various doctors and decided upon a course of therapy that included hormone treatments in November and radiation beginning in January 2000. However, before that happened, I talked with a physician who suggested that a visit to the Paracelsus Clinic might be more beneficial than radiation. So I scheduled a three-week visit to Paracelsus in March.

I completed a course of neural therapy, as well as magnetic therapy, which is a treatment of about 20 minutes, during which magnetic fields surround the area of the cancer. Localized heat therapy was also part of my regimen, and I received ozone treatments as well. I had lots of dental work done, including removal of mercury fillings and three teeth. I made a follow-up visit to Paracelsus in early 2001.

I continue to consult with my personal physicians, with an oncologist who is neutral regarding a patient's choice of conventional versus alternative methods, and with a homeopathic physician here in New Mexico. I am on high intravenous doses of vitamin C, as well as other homeopathic medications that neutralize acidity and promote an environment in which the cancer cannot grow.

As a result of all this, I am healthy and active, and I never had to have the radiation.

## Arnold "Buff" Chace, 54, *businessman, Providence, R.I.* (*bladder cancer*)

In November 1998, I noticed blood in my urine and went to a urologist for a diagnosis. Under general anesthesia, I underwent an examination of the urethra, during which a tumor was discovered and excised for analysis. This proved to be the source of blood in the urine, and I was diagnosed with transitional cell carcinoma, a cancer for which, if it reappeared, the outlook was not good. The literature suggests that this type of cancer has a 75 percent chance of recurring.

When I asked how and why I might have contracted the cancer, the doctors asked if I worked in a tannery or smoked. When I answered no to both questions, they said they did not know. Their best advice was to repeat the diagnostic procedure every three months to check for recurrence, something that I still do today.

However, I was not satisfied and wanted to know what steps I could take to prevent recurrence. I was familiar with Margie Baldwin at the Marion Institute and was aware of the situation with her son, Nathaniel.* I knew that after Nathaniel visited the Paracelsus Clinic and Dr. Thomas Rau, his condition improved significantly. So I did some research on Paracelsus and because of their interest in why things occur, I decided that this was my type of place.

I went to Paracelsus in January 1999 for a two-week stay. I was found to have heavy-metal toxicity, as well as an immune system that was compromised and very weak. Dr. Rau initiated a number of natural therapies and made many adjustments in the regimen to ensure that they were effective. I also had all of my mercury amalgam fillings removed and replaced.

---

* See "Nathaniel's story," in the Preface.

With the help of Paracelsus, I adopted a different approach to diet — mostly vegetarian — that would promote "flushing" my system of all the heavy metals. Dr. Rau calls it "changing the milieu" to one that promotes better health.

There were also regular heat treatments, mistletoe injections, colon-cleansing procedures, ozone treatments, and neural therapy, including injections into the bladder. Observing the principles of the meridian system, Dr. Rau identified a splitting tooth that related to the bladder — the site of the cancer. The tooth was injected as a way of rejuvenating it.

I have taken various vitamins and minerals and make a point to exercise to produce a sweat, which helps rid the body of toxins.

It's interesting to note that mercury levels in my blood have actually increased, which just indicates how much mercury was in the tissue and needs to be expelled.

The bottom line is that since my first visit to Paracelsus, there has been no recurrence of the cancer. I am totally sold on this approach to health care, and I am particularly impressed by Dr. Rau's open approach and willingness to employ whatever works. He does not follow a strict approach to treatment, is not set in his ways at all, and is into results.

Because this holistic approach to medicine addresses the psychological component of disease as well, I have taken steps to change the ways in which I deal with stress.

I have been so impressed that I have referred several family members and friends to Paracelsus for everything from hyperthyroidism and an oversized wisdom tooth to breast cancer and other cancers. I really believe that this is a very beneficial approach to one's health.

## Kathrin Scheel Ungerleider, *51, painting conservator, New York, N.Y. (breast cancer)*

My recovery from breast cancer, diagnosed in 1998 one year after my husband's death from cancer, was difficult. The tumor had been found early and was treated conventionally with surgical excision and radiation.

Although my prognosis was good, my health spiraled downward. Major problems occurred each year, ranging from extreme fatigue, impaired equilibrium, unnecessary surgery on the other breast for a suspected tumor, to months of severe panic and depression. Finally, I followed a trusted friend's advice and went to the Paracelsus Clinic in August of 2001, as a patient of Dr. Rau.

Since then my health and state of mind have begun to stabilize and take a decisive turn for the better. Although being a patient with a life-threatening illness is never easy, I immediately felt that here was an integrated, holistic response to my symptoms, which before had been viewed as unrelated.

I encountered a non-alarmist, nurturing atmosphere, where suffering and uncertainty were "held" very differently from the way I had experienced previously. In addition, the many avenues of inquiry into the psychic and spiritual underpinnings of my condition offered at the clinic awakened my interest and soon trust in my own life's strange path. And, as I started to feel better, I recognized the opportunity offered by this illness and found support for deep change. Slowly, during many subsequent visits, I began to gain knowledge of and confidence in Paracelsus Biological Medicine, which I had been unfamiliar with.

Here was an alternative to the — with exceptions of course — crazed, fragmented, and dogmatic response to complex health problems that conventional medicine offers nowadays. Finding it completely worthwhile to put my trust in this paradigm, I am, by doing so, furthering an excellent alternative approach to healing and health maintenance.

I believe that we, as patients, need Paracelsus Biological Medicine, while also having the privilege and duty to strengthen its base by learning more about it and spreading the word.

When allopathic medicine — generally portrayed as unquestionable — offers insufficient help, the patient is challenged not to accept that. For me, rising to this challenge means learning to trust myself and taking responsibility for my health care decisions. Paracelsus Biological Medicine as practiced at Lustmühle is an integral part of my return to physical and emotional health.

### Jens Rune Sortland, *52, engineer, Sandes, Norway* (*chronic pharyngitis and laryngitis, high mercury levels*)

When I was about 18 years old, I had a constant sore throat that never seemed to go away — like a flu or cold. I am now 52, and over the past 10 years my symptoms have become significantly worse. In addition to my sore throat and night sweats, I also experienced pain in my left leg and lower back.

In 2006, I had surgery to remove a disc prolapse in my lower-lumbar back, which resulted in an infection in the adjacent vertebrae. A massive broad-spectrum antibiotic was prescribed, because the bacteria was never isolated or identified. Although I did have a period of improvement, I never recovered completely from this. For the past six months I have been unable to work or participate in normal physical activities, despite my eating healthy foods and exercising regularly.

The many doctors and natural medicine practitioners that I have seen over the years were unable to find any specific problem or treatment for my condition. The usual response was everything looks good, tests were fine, and I should be ok. When I arrived at the Paracelsus Clinic, I was diagnosed with amalgam poisoning, which in turn weakened my immune defense system and caused food allergies. And in his Darkfield, Dr. Rau also found "cell wall deficient bacteria" which he treated with Sanum remedies and neural therapies. During the two weeks stay, I had a remarkable improvement in my health condition. This is the first time in my life that I have received a medical treatment that appears to work on the symptoms that have bothered me for so long!

After returning home from the Paracelsus Clinic, I continue to take the prescribed medicines and follow the dietary instructions given to me. I have returned to work full-time and am on the road to recovery.

# Conclusion
# Is Paracelsus Biological Medicine for Me?

WHEN YOU ASSUME THE ROLE of patient, you need to feel as comfortable and confident as possible with your choice of practitioner and methods of diagnosis and treatment. Consideration of appropriate health care choices is an intensely personal journey for everyone, from the selection of over-the-counter medications at a retail drugstore to decisions regarding treatment for debilitating and life-threatening diseases.

Paracelsus Biological Medicine (PBM) is perhaps not the answer for everybody, but its philosophies and principles are sound and provide worthwhile health care solutions for people worldwide. The fact that you have read this guidebook suggests that you have taken the first step toward making a commitment to a deeper level of personal health care that can generate rewards for a lifetime — hopefully, a longer lifetime.

We hope the overview we have presented here will help you make informed decisions about your own health care, beginning right now.

Please utilize the resources in the appendices to find additional information about PBM and types of alternative health care, or contact the Paracelsus Biological Medicine Network (PBMN) at the Marion Institute to learn more about the Paracelsus Clinic in Switzerland or a PBM practitioner near you.

# Appendix A
# About the Marion Institute:
# Creating Deep and Positive Change

FOUNDED IN 1992 and located in Marion, Massachusetts, the Marion Institute seeks to unite people who want to heal themselves — and the planet — by encouraging a deeper understanding of the past, a dynamic experience of the present, and a passionate vision of a healthy future. We believe in the interdependence of all life and the critical balance necessary for a sustainable future. To this end, the Marion Institute is an organization that seeks to address the root causes of problems through a comprehensive systemic approach that identifies related problems and then designs an initiative that addresses multiple problems simultaneously.

The Marion Institute seeks to identify and promote the world's most ground-breaking innovators in the realms of the environment, health, business, spirituality, sustainable farming — and beyond — in an effort to advance and help others to replicate their work.

Just as nature itself is diverse, the Marion Institute encompasses a variety of diverse programs that inspire a deeper look at the unique yet interconnected elements that sustain human life. The Marion Institute supports the following programs: the Paracelsus Biological Medicine Network (health and healing); Natural Capital Institute (socially responsible investing and business); Metahistory

> "When there were few who believed in what we were doing here, in the Green Belt Movement — when our little tree-planting movement often suffered repression, violence and jail time — the Marion Institute always stood by me. The Institute has generously helped raise financial support and awareness for the work of the Green Belt Movement. But more importantly, they have been a deep source of inspiration, emotional support and sustenance for me. Every tree needs water at its roots. It would not have been possible to plant all these trees and hope without the support and friends and partners like the Marion Institute."
>
> - Wangari Maathai
> 2004 Nobel Peace
> Prize Winner

(spirituality: belief-driving behavior); ZERI Learning (sustainability education); Gaviotas (carbon offset initiative); and Serendipity projects (diverse programs and projects created by passionate folks); Bioneers by the Bay: Connecting for Change (annual conference to connect society with system thinkers and innovators); and How on Earth (local food movement and sustainable farming).

The Marion Institute strives to engage the widest possible number of people and to inspire them to create *deep and positive change* in the world and in themselves.

## Paracelsus Biological Medicine Network (PBMN)

In 1997, the Marion Institute joined with the Paracelsus Clinic in Switzerland to create the Paracelsus Biological Medicine Network (PBMN), dedicated to the vision of healing embodied by Paracelsus Biological Medicine.

Our mission is to make Paracelsus Biological Medicine available to the vast numbers of Americans who are bewildered by and dissatisfied with the conventional medical options presented to them. The PBMN educates patients, trains practitioners, coordinates referrals, cultivates the ever-growing community of PBM patients, helps

"For more than 10 years now, the Paracelsus Biological Medicine Network has enjoyed a tremendously productive partnership with the Marion Institute. The Institute team offers us much more than logistical administrative support. They bring a deep dedication to the holistic and spiritual aspects of Paracelsus Biological Medicine. The Marion Institute has also worked to craft a network of practitioners and patients for PBMN — in North America and around the world. In short, with their tireless work and endless passion, the Marion Institute is responsible for building critical awareness and support for this most essential alternative approach to health and healing."

- Dr. Thomas Rau

organize publications (e.g. *The Swiss Secret to Optimal Health*), and creates strategies to disseminate this invaluable information.

Long available in Europe, biological medicine is now delivering benefits to countless North Americans, offering a comprehensive approach to medical care that enables individuals to take responsibility for their health and healing throughout life.

We invite you to learn more about the PBMN and the Marion Institute. Our supplementary materials provide comprehensive descriptions of our activities.

Paracelsus Biological Medicine Network
Marion Institute
202 Spring Street
Marion, MA 02738

Phone: 508.748.0816
Fax: 508.748.1976

www.marioninstitute.org
www.pbmn.org
info@pbmn.org

# Appendix B
# About the Paracelsus Clinic

The Paracelsus Clinic in Lustmühle, Switzerland, was founded in 1958 as a center for health and well-being based on the principles of natural healing. Since then, it has integrated and adapted to the evolving models of biological and holistic medicine and dentistry. Growing patient demand led to the establishment of Paracelsus Clinic Al Ronc, which offers inpatient care, in southern Switzerland in 2001.

The Paracelsus Clinic Lustmühle is the only outpatient clinic in Switzerland in which the full range of biological medicine is combined with conventional and state-of-the-art therapies designed to help balance and restore the overall regulation of the body's systems. This unique model also includes the integration of holistic dentistry. The clinic assists patients to secure accommodations in nearby hotels.

At Lustmühle, a team of more than 80 motivated people work closely together: eight physicians, three dentists, a team of therapists and nurses, pharmacists, consultants from different scientific specializations, medical assistants, dental technicians, and administrative assistants. Thus, a combination of treatments can be offered to meet the differing needs of patients. In nearly all cases of acute and chronic disease, the patient can be either treated or advised successfully.

The clinic also serves as an educational resource foundation for holistic medicine, offering further education to doctors, dentists, non-medical practitioners, pharmacists, and other therapists.

## Treating acute and chronic disease, including cancer

Who goes to Paracelsus?

In addition to those who visit the clinic for preventive and health-maintenance reasons, patients from all over the world choose Paracelsus because of its reputation for successfully treating many different diseases, including cancer, and very often without surgery, chemotherapy, or radiation. Patients with breast and prostate cancer have had some of the most positive results.

Chronic conditions like arthritis, asthma, allergies, endometriosis, and autoimmune diseases such as multiple sclerosis, Lyme disease, and Parkinson's are also commonly treated.

The clinic is also well-known for its diagnostic check-ups. A broad variety of fine energetic diagnostic tools can identify illness symptoms before they advance and need intensive care.

## Importance of dentistry

Dental treatment is a key factor in this Paracelsus Biological Medicine system, as extensive study has found that the teeth, as well as the jaw, are frequently the cause for disease located elsewhere in the body. The dental clinic offers a wide variety of diagnostic methods, which make it unique. It is one of only three clinics in Europe that use a Cavitat medical imaging device to detect interference fields using ultrasound. Thermography and other fine energetic examination methods are used to show infections, disturbance foci, and joint displacements.

The dental clinic is extremely conscious about the materials used for dental replacements. Our dentists work exclusively with metal-free materials. Ceramic (Zirkonium) implants replace the more common titanium implants, which can cause toxic problems and intolerances. The latest introduction in this field is the Zirkonium two-piece implant.

Another focus of the clinic is amalgam removal and cleansing. The clinic's applied techniques avoid the dangerous effects of the removal, which can lead to severe side effects. A newly developed ozone-generator is used for the removal of bacterial infections.

## On-site pharmacy

The on-site pharmacy at Paracelsus carries a complete range of biological supplements and medicines.

## Paracelsus Clinic Al Ronc

The Paracelsus Clinic Al Ronc is situated in Castaneda, high above the Calanca Valley and 800 meters above sea level. Built in 1986, the clinic was completely modernized in 2001. Since then, this biological health center works closely with the Paracelsus Clinic Lustmühle.

The clinic's modern building, nestled within a stand of chestnut trees, is surrounded by the flora typically found in the southern part of Switzerland. Breathtaking nature trails invite guests to stroll in the untouched Calanca Valley or to visit Santa Maria, an idyllic mountain hamlet above the clinic. Guests who prefer not to ramble can enjoy the peace and quiet of the park at Al Ronc and dream away the day in these perfect surroundings.

In this restorative setting, guests are invited to focus on what really matters in life through medical examinations, treatments, and an organic/vegetarian eating plan designed to take the strain off the body. A visit to the Paracelsus Clinic Al Ronc is a journey into health that can have a preventive effect or can reverse chronic health problems that have existed for years.

The clinic offers treatments for individual illnesses as well as special theme weeks, such as Dr. Rau's Intensive Al Ronc Week, the Paracelsus heavy metal detoxification plan, burn-out syndrome, the Paracelsus liver and gall bladder plan, and the Paracelsus fasting plan.

## Cost and other considerations

Both clinics are operated by the same management. The optimum duration of a clinic visit is from two-to-four weeks. The cost varies according to the amount and kind of dental work and supplements prescribed, as well as travel considerations and type of accommodations, which the clinics can help to arrange.

The total cost of your visit may range from $5,000 to $25,000. For inquiries and registration, visit www.paracelsus.ch, www.alronc.ch, or www.pbmn.org.

## Does health insurance cover any of the consultations or treatments?

It depends on the state you live in and your insurance plan. A few states and some health plans are expanding coverage to include some types of alternative health care. The clinic does not work directly with U.S. health insurance providers, so if you do have coverage, you would pay out of pocket for the expenses and then submit to your insurance company for reimbursement. It is advisable to contact your insurance company prior to your visits.

## Is there a comparable clinic in the United States?

The Paracelsus Clinic is unique, in that all of the services are in one facility, including specialty diagnostic equipment, dental services, treatment capabilities, and a pharmacy. There are some individual doctors in North America practicing some aspects of Paracelsus Biological Medicine, but none is able at this time to provide a complete array of services and comprehensive work-ups. Please call the Paracelsus Biological Medicine Network (PBMN) at 508.748.0816 for names of practitioners in your area.

## How long is the wait to get an appointment?

It varies, depending on the season, the doctors' schedules, and which doctors you need to see. In general, it can take between one and four months to arrange for your first stay. It can take up to 20 working days to get an appointment date or phone consultation.

## Will I get to see Dr. Rau?

Dr. Rau has limited openings for new patients. He always sees patients in conjunction with another doctor. However, his schedule is booked well in advance. He has several colleagues who have worked with him for many years, and provide comparable care to Dr. Rau. All doctors at the clinic have trained and worked with Dr. Rau, and are fully qualified Paracelsus Biological Medicine physicians. You will see your assigned doctor on your first day and many times during your stay.

## How can I prepare for my trip?

We advise you to familiarize yourself as much as possible with the principles of Paracelsus Biological Medicine. Check our websites www.pbmn.org or www.paracelsus.ch for an overview of the philosophy and more in-depth information. We highly recommend that you also read Dr. Rau's book, *The Swiss Secret to Optimal Health*.

## What can I expect when I arrive at the clinic?

All of the staff at both the Paracelsus and Al Ronc clinics speak English. There will be a schedule of your first-day appointments and an information packet waiting for you at the hotel. Review that carefully. All the staff at the clinic and the Santis Hotel are very helpful. Don't be afraid to ask your questions. One of your first appointments will be with the patient coordinator at the clinic, who will go over everything with you, and is always available to address your questions and concerns.

## What about food?

If you stay at the Santis Hotel in Lustmühle, your breakfast will be provided, and dinner is offered. All meals follow Dr. Rau's recommended diet. The Culinarium Restaurant is next to the clinic, which offers choices also following the clinic diet plan. There are also several very nice restaurants in Teufen and St. Gallen which are delicious and vegetarian. The clinic can provide you with some names.

There is a nutritionist on staff to go over your diet with you. Ask for an appointment in advance.

# Glossary

**ALLOPATHIC**  System of therapeutics in which diseases are treated by producing a condition that is incompatible with or antagonistic to the disease and its symptoms; conventional Western medicine is said to be allopathic.

**AYURVEDIC MEDICINE**  Theory that suggests that diseases of the body are caused by stresses in the awareness, or consciousness, of the individual; ayurvedic treatments include yoga-related body postures, breathing exercises, meditative techniques, special diets, and herbal remedies.

**BIOLOGICAL MEDICINE**  Holistic approach to health and wellness that allows the human body to maximize its own innate healing powers; combines traditional healing practices with modern, noninvasive diagnostic and treatment methods.

**BODYWORK**  Variety of techniques that promote relaxation and treat certain ailments, especially musculoskeletal disorders. Treatments include massage, movement awareness, structural realignment, and energy balancing.

**HOLISTIC**  Approach to medicine that assumes that the human being is a functioning system operating in a "state of wholeness"; holistic medicine views all aspects of an individual — physical, mental, emotional, and spiritual — as interrelated.

**HOMEOPATHY**  Therapeutic system in which diseases are treated by substances that can cause symptoms of disease in a healthy person but that, when administered in minute doses, can cure the same symptoms.

KINESTHESIA  The science of movement; in biological medicine, refers to movement and angles of joints that may be indicative of disease.

NATUROPATHY  System of medicine that treats health conditions by utilizing the body's inherent, natural ability to heal; diet, lifestyle, work, and personal history are all considered when determining a treatment regimen.

NEURAL THERAPY  Injection of homeopathic remedies into the body's acupuncture points.

OSTEOPATHY  Medical discipline that focuses on addressing problems in the musculoskeletal system to correct and improve the general functioning of the body.

THERMOGRAPHY  Diagnostic technique that utilizes a thermalized (temperature-sensitive) wand, or thermister, to record skin temperature at 181 points on the body, first at standard room temperature, then at a lower temperature; responses provide feedback on functioning of organs and systems.

TRADITIONAL CHINESE MEDICINE  Ancient system of holistic health care that uses a variety of treatments including acupressure, acupuncture, herbal therapies, and massage, along with health-sustaining energetic body movement such as tai chi.

# Resource List

## Books

*Between Heaven and Earth: A Guide to Chinese Medicine*
Harriet Beinfield and Efrem Korngold
Paperback
ISBN: 0345379748
Random House
1992

*The Complete Book of Chinese Health & Healing*
Daniel Reid and Dexter Chow
Paperback
ISBN: 1570620717
Shambhala
1995

*Conscious Eating*
Gabriel Cousens, MD
Paperback
ISBN: 1556432852
North Atlantic Books
2000

*Everybody's Guide to Homeopathic Medicines*
Stephen Cummings, MD, and Dana Ullman, MPH
Paperback
ISBN: 0874778433
Putnam Publishing Group
1997

*Healing with Whole Foods: Oriental Traditions and
    Modern Nutrition*
Paul Pitchford
Paperback
ISBN: 1556432208
North Atlantic Books
1996

*Homeopathy: Medicine of the New Man*
George Vithoulkas
Paperback
Simon & Schuster
ISBN: 0671763288
1985

*Radical Healing: Integrating the World's Great Therapeutic
    Traditions to Create a New Transformative Medicine*
Rudolph M. Ballantine
Paperback
ISBN: 0609804847
Crown
2000

*Reclaiming the Wisdom of the Body: A Personal Guide to Chinese Medicine*
Sandra Hill
Paperback
ISBN: 0806520736
Carol
1999

*Root Canal Cover-Up*
George E. Meinig
Charlene Koonce and Mark Lovendale (Editors)
Paperback
ISBN: 0945196199
Bion
1994

*The Swiss Secret to Optimal Health*
Thomas Rau, MD, with Susan Wyler
Hardcover
Berkley Books
ISBN: 9780425213933
2007

*Theory and Practice of Biological Medicine*
David A. Edwards, MD, HMD
Paperback
ISBN: 0964732505
MG Reprographics
1995

*Tooth Truth*
Frank J. Jerome, DDS
Paperback
ISBN: 1890035130
New Century Press
2001


*The Toxic Time Bomb: Can the Mercury in Your Dental Fillings
    Poison You?*
Sam Ziff
Foreword by Jeffery Bland
Paperback
ISBN: 0943358248
Aurora Press
1985


*Uninformed Consent: The Hidden Dangers in Dental Care*
Hal A. Huggins and Thomas E. Levy
Paperback
ISBN: 1571741178
Hampton Roads
1998


*Whole-Body Dentistry: Discover the Missing Piece to
    Better Health*
Mark A. Breiner with Foreword by Denise Dolence
Introduction by Robert C. Atkins
Paperback
ISBN: 0967844304
Quantum Health Press
1999

The
Dr. Rau's Diet for
Whole Body Healing

# SWISS

# SECRET

## to Optimal Health

**Build a better body, cell by cell**

# Thomas Rau, M.D.

with Susan Wyler

Foreword by Dr. Mark Hyman